DRUGS: SHATTER THE MYTHS

What does the National Institute on Drug Abuse do?

NIDA is part of the National Institutes of Health. We are the largest supporter of the world's research on drug abuse and addiction. Our goal is to better understand who uses drugs and why, and how drugs work in the brain and body, so we can develop and test new ways to prevent and treat drug abuse and addiction.

This publication is in the public domain and may be used or reproduced in its entirety without permission from NIDA. Citation of the source is appreciated.

NIH Publication No. 15-7589
Printed October 2010
Revised April 2011, July 2013, March 2015

Table of Contents

- **4** Marijuana
- **8** Peer Pressure
- **12** Alcohol
- **14** Medical Consequences
- **19** Rx Drugs
- **22** Drugs & Your Brain
- **26** Treatment

TOPIC
Marijuana

Is marijuana ADDICTIVE?

Yes. The chances of becoming addicted to marijuana or any drug are different for each person. For marijuana, around **1 in 11** people who use it become addicted. Could **you** be *that* one?

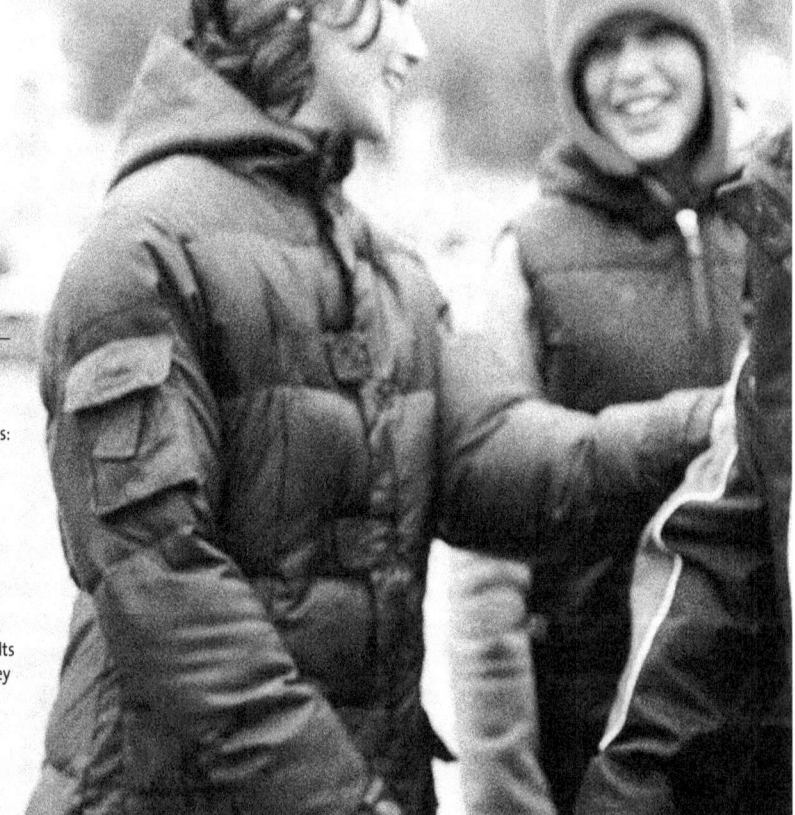

Anthony J, Warner LA, Kessler RC. Comparative epidemiology of dependence on tobacco, alcohol, controlled substances, and inhalants: basic findings from the National Comorbidity Survey. *Exp Clin Psychopharmacol.* 1994;2:244–268.

Lopez-Quintero C, Pérez de los Cobos J, Hasin DS, et al. Probability and predictors of transition from first use to dependence on nicotine, alcohol, cannabis, and cocaine: results of the National Epidemiologic Survey on Alcohol and Related Conditions (NESARC). *Drug Alcohol Depend.* 2011;115(1–2):120–130.

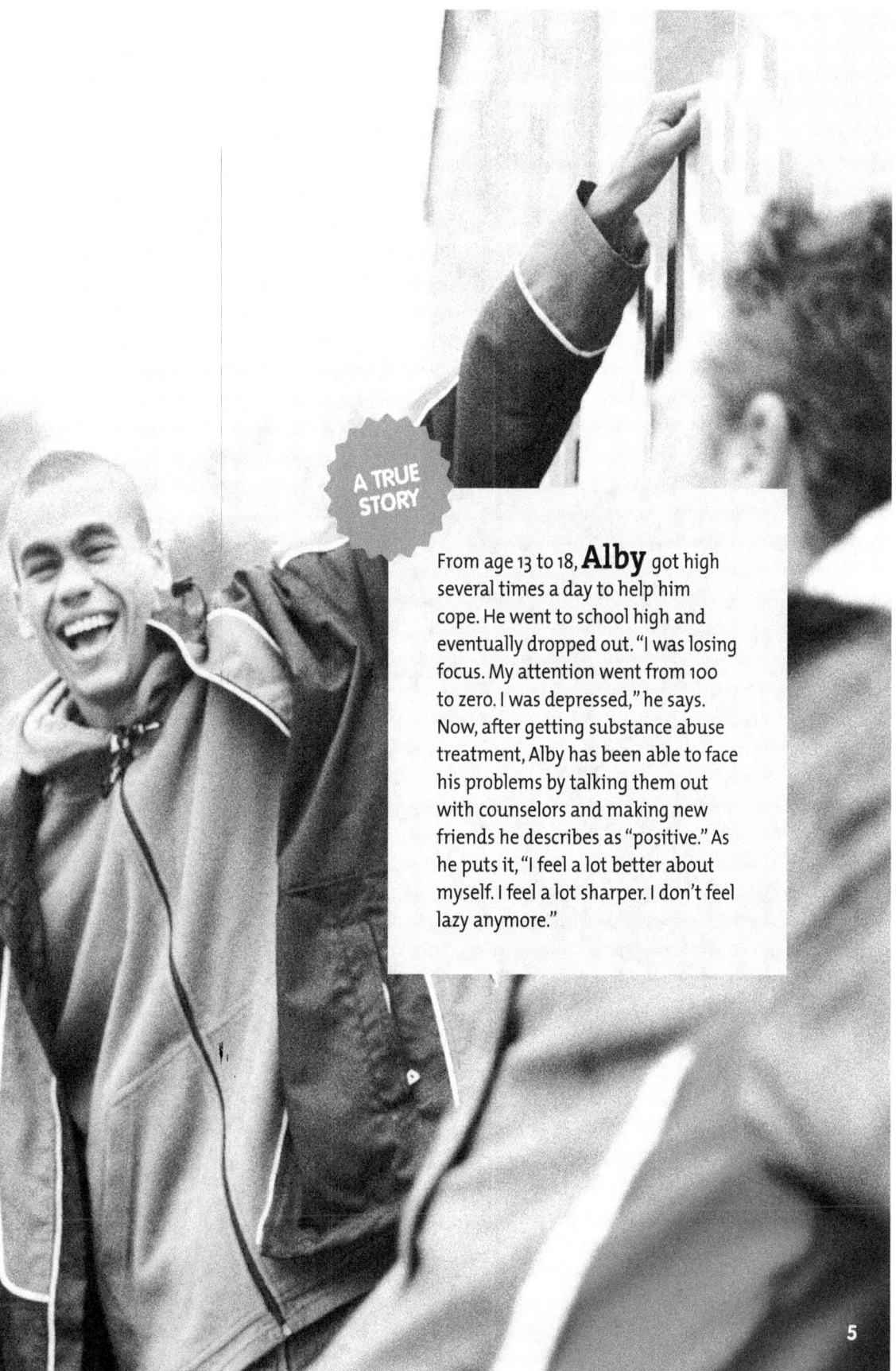

A TRUE STORY

From age 13 to 18, **Alby** got high several times a day to help him cope. He went to school high and eventually dropped out. "I was losing focus. My attention went from 100 to zero. I was depressed," he says. Now, after getting substance abuse treatment, Alby has been able to face his problems by talking them out with counselors and making new friends he describes as "positive." As he puts it, "I feel a lot better about myself. I feel a lot sharper. I don't feel lazy anymore."

FACT

IF YOU SMOKE MARIJUANA A LOT IN YOUR TEENS, YOU COULD LOSE IQ POINTS THAT YOU MIGHT NEVER GET BACK.

Meier MH, Caspi A, Ambler A, et al. Persistent cannabis users show neuropsychological decline from childhood to midlife. *Proc Natl Acad Sci USA*. 2012;109:E2657-2664.

QUIZ

Why isn't smoked marijuana a safe medicine?
- A. You can't be sure what chemicals are in it.
- B. Smoking anything can hurt your lungs.
- C. It affects your thinking skills.
- D. It alters your motor skills, making you an unsafe driver.
- E. All of the above

Which of these webs is made by a spider that is NOT on drugs?

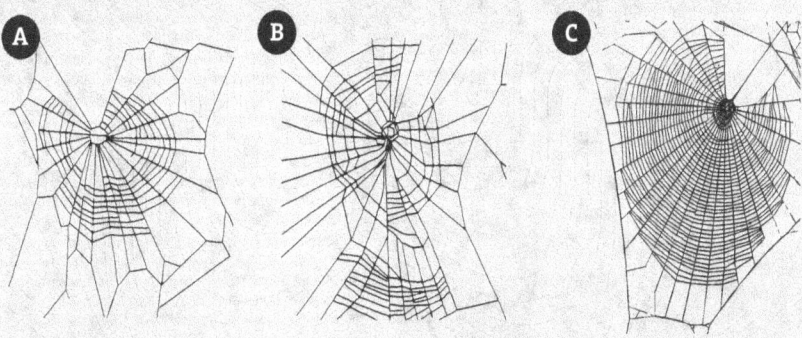

"Spice" (also known as K-2):
- A. Is considered to be a "fake marijuana"
- B. Has put people in emergency rooms with vomiting, confusion, and hallucinations
- C. Is abused mainly by smoking
- D. All of the above

ANSWERS: E. All of the above, C. No Drugs, D. All of the above

Product Placement

Product Placement

A lot of teens ask us about **peer pressure**, or why people do things that can hurt them just to fit in.

TOPIC
Peer Pressure

Why do people

SMOKE

when they know it's so bad for them?

Maybe they smoke because they can't stop. People start smoking for different reasons, but most keep doing it because of one reason—they are addicted to nicotine.

Product Placement

DID YOU KNOW? Research says that teens who see a lot of smoking in movies are more likely to start smoking themselves. Sometimes characters smoke to look edgy and rebellious; but sometimes it's just about "product placement"—the tobacco industry trying to get into your head and your pockets.

U.S. Department of Health and Human Services. *Preventing Tobacco Use Among Youth and Young Adults: A Report of the Surgeon General.* Atlanta, GA: U.S. Department of Health and Human Services, Centers for Disease Control and Prevention, National Center for Chronic Disease Prevention and Health Promotion, Office on Smoking and Health; 2012.

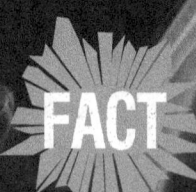

MOST PEOPLE WHO SMOKE STARTED BEFORE AGE 18.

U.S. Department of Health and Human Services. *Preventing Tobacco Use Among Youth and Young Adults: A Report of the Surgeon General.* Atlanta, GA: U.S. Department of Health and Human Services, Centers for Disease Control and Prevention, National Center for Chronic Disease Prevention and Health Promotion, Office on Smoking and Health; 2012.

QUIZ

Smokeless tobacco does not cause cancer.
- A. True, it is the tar in cigarettes that causes lung cancer, emphysema, and bronchial disorders.
- B. False, smokeless tobacco (such as chewing tobacco and snuff) increases the risk of cancer, especially oral cancers.

How many Americans die from diseases associated with tobacco use each year?
- A. About 1,500
- B. About 13,200
- C. About 50,500
- D. About 480,000

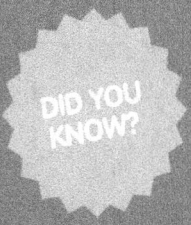

E-Cigarettes

E-cigarettes contain nicotine — the addictive drug in tobacco cigarettes — and other chemicals that may be harmful.

More teens use e-cigarettes than tobacco cigarettes. Scientists have just started to research the health effects of e-cigarettes, but we do know one thing: users will inhale the same nicotine they get from a regular cigarette.

U.S. Department of Health and Human Services. *The Health Consequences of Smoking — 50 Years of Progress. A Report of the Surgeon General.* Atlanta, GA: U.S. Department of Health and Human Services, Centers for Disease Control and Prevention, National Center for Chronic Disease Prevention and Health Promotion, Office on Smoking and Health; 2014.

ANSWERS: B. False, D. About 480,000

TOPIC
Alcohol

DRINKING
and driving can add up to tragic endings. In the U.S., about 4,300 people under age 21 die each year from injuries caused by underage drinking, more than 35 percent in car crashes.

Centers for Disease Control and Prevention. Alcohol Related Disease Impact (ARDI) application, 2013. Available at http://apps.nccd.cdc.gov/DACH_ARDI/Default.aspx.

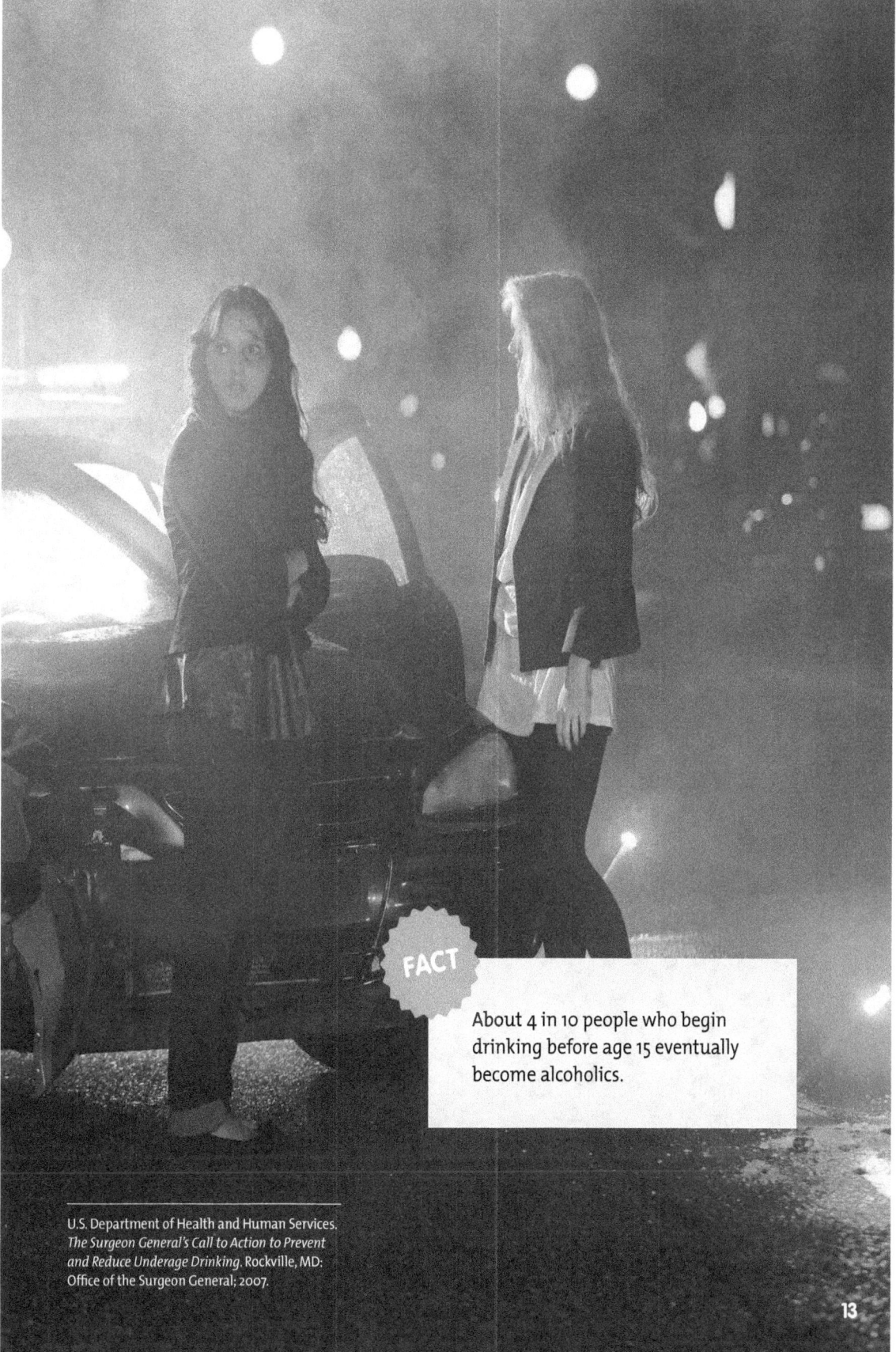

FACT

About 4 in 10 people who begin drinking before age 15 eventually become alcoholics.

U.S. Department of Health and Human Services. *The Surgeon General's Call to Action to Prevent and Reduce Underage Drinking*. Rockville, MD: Office of the Surgeon General; 2007.

TOPIC
Medical Consequences

HIV
Getting HIV from unprotected sex

When you can't think straight because you're drunk or high, you may forget to play it safe. Kim did—read her story at:
www.hiv.drugabuse.gov/english/webisodes/theParty.html

Meth

Meth reduces the amount of protective saliva around the teeth. People who use meth also tend to drink a lot of sugary soda, neglect personal hygiene, grind their teeth, and clench their jaws—all of which can cause what's known as "meth mouth."

Meth users sometimes hallucinate that insects are creeping on top of or underneath their skin (called formication). The person will pick or scratch their skin, trying to get rid of the imaginary "crank bugs." Soon their face and arms are covered with open sores that can get infected. See more at: www.teens.drugabuse.gov/drug-facts/methamphetamine-meth

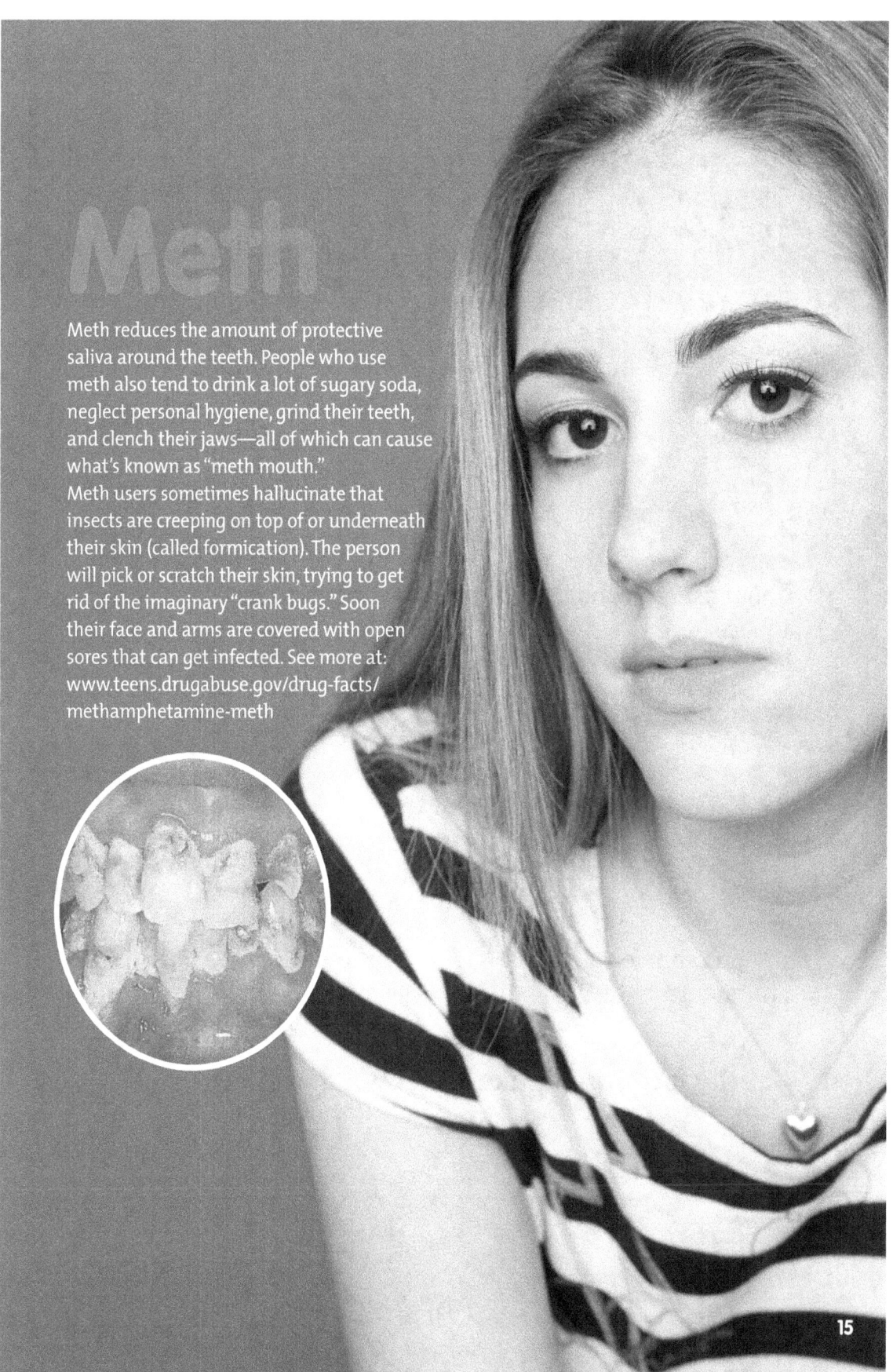

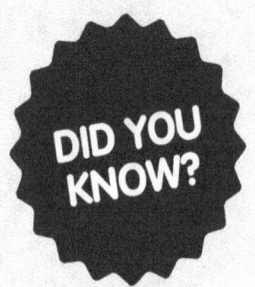

DID YOU KNOW?

You are getting bombarded with messages about drugs in songs and movies. A 2008 study of popular music found that about

1 in 3 songs said something about drug, alcohol, or tobacco use.

3 in 4 rap songs said something about drug, alcohol, or tobacco use.

And of the top 100 movies over a 9-year period, more than

7 in 10 movies showed characters smoking.

1 in 3 movies showed people getting drunk.

Get the facts, and make your own decisions.

Primack BA, Dalton MA, Carroll MV, Agarwal AA, Fine MJ. Content analysis of tobacco, alcohol, and other drugs in popular music. Arch Pediatr Adolesc Med. 2008;162(2):169–174.

Tickle JJ, Beach ML, Dalton ML. Tobacco, alcohol, and other risk behaviors in film: how well do MPAA ratings distinguish content? J Health Commun. 2009;14(8):756–767.

Tobacco

Wrinkles, bad breath, yellow teeth, wheezing, stinky clothes?...Let me at those cigarettes!

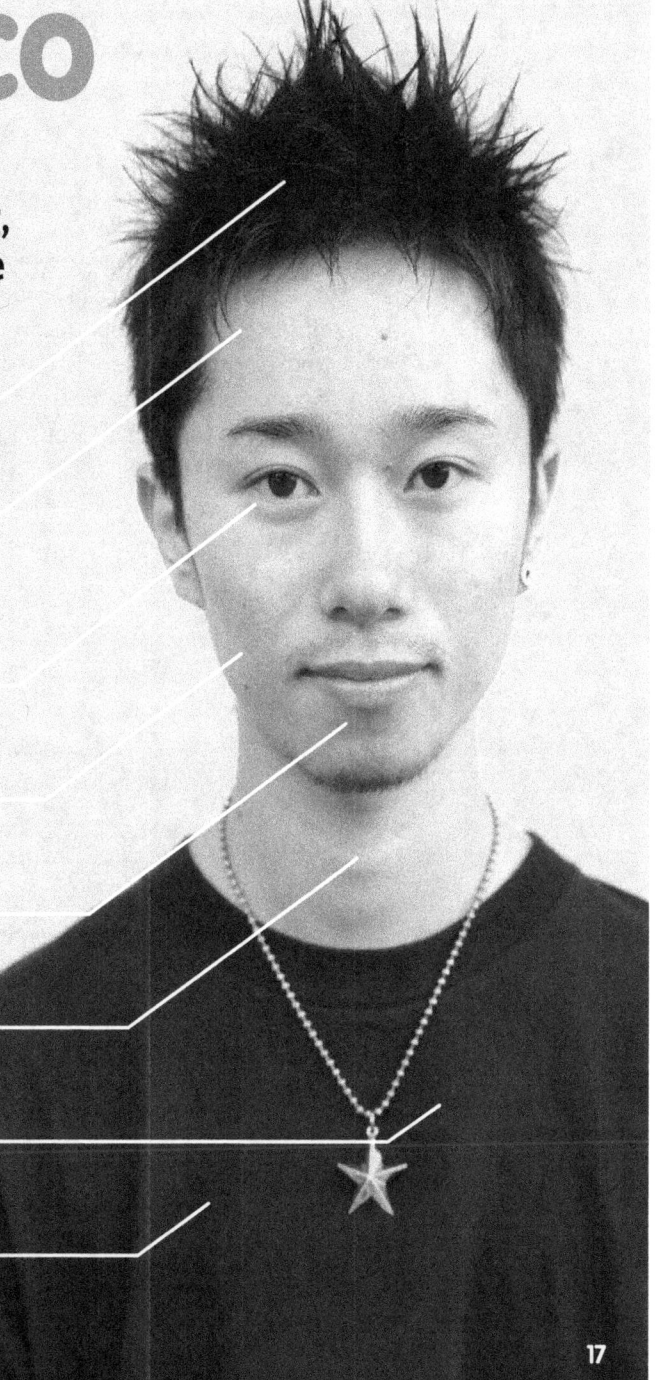

ADDICTION

SKIN DAMAGE

CATARACTS

WRINKLES

MOUTH CANCERS

THROAT CANCER

HEART DISEASE

LUNG DISEASE

Q&A

What is Vicodin?

Vicodin is a medication prescribed to relieve pain. When taken as prescribed it can be very effective, helping people recover from surgery, for example. But it is from the same class of drugs as heroin and can be dangerous if used to get high.

FACT

More people die from prescription pain reliever overdoses (like Vicodin and OxyContin) than from heroin and cocaine combined.

Centers for Disease Control and Prevention. *Prescription Painkiller Overdoses in the US.* www.cdc.gov/vitalsigns/PainkillerOverdoses/index.html. Updated: November 1, 2011. Accessed: February 18, 2015.

TOPIC
Rx Drugs

A lot of you have asked: how can

PRESCRIPTION (RX) DRUGS

be harmful when they're prescribed by doctors? Prescription drugs aren't bad—they totally help a lot of people. It really depends on the *who, how,* and *why* of it.

- *Who* were they prescribed for (you or someone else)?
- *How* are you taking them (as prescribed or not)?
- *Why* (to get well or to get high)?

Some teens abuse stimulants thinking it will improve their grades; in fact, it may do just the opposite!

FACT

RX DRUG ABUSE IS DRUG ABUSE.

QUIZ

It's safe to use prescription drugs when:
- A. You've checked out WebMD and know what you are doing
- B. You've taken them before for another problem
- C. They are prescribed for you by a doctor for a current problem
- D. Your mom gave them to you from her prescription
- E. All of the above

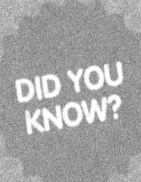
DID YOU KNOW?

Mixing pills with other drugs or with alcohol really increases your risk of death from accidental overdose.

Abuse of prescription stimulants like Ritalin and Adderall can cause serious health problems, including panic attacks, seizures, and heart attacks.

ANSWERS: C. They are prescribed for you by a doctor for a current problem.

TOPIC
Drugs & Your Brain

You know they make you

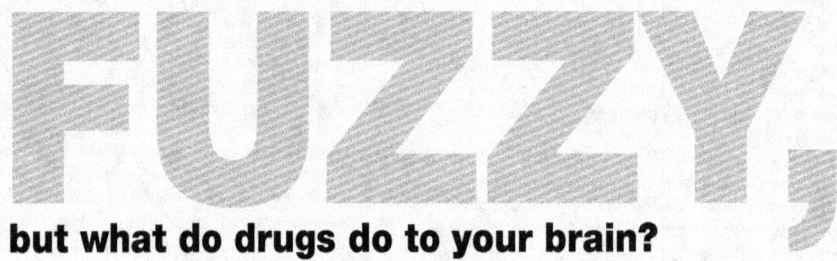

but what do drugs do to your brain?

Different drugs do different things. But they *all* affect the brain—that's why drugs make you feel high, low, speeded up, or slowed down, or see things that aren't there.

DID YOU KNOW? Repeated drug use can reset the brain's pleasure meter, so that without the drug, you feel hopeless and sad. Eventually, everyday fun stuff like spending time with friends or playing with your dog doesn't make you happy anymore.

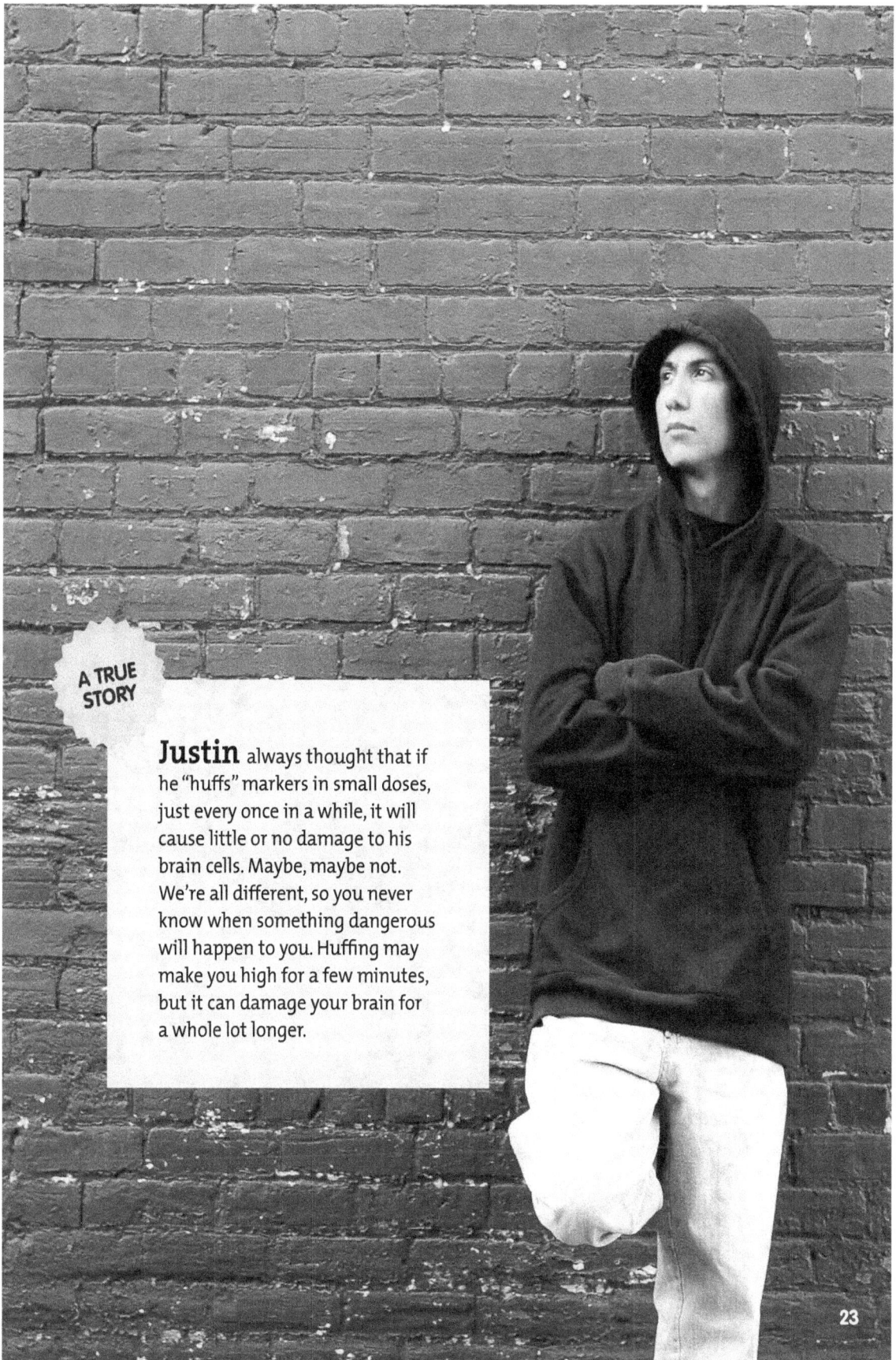

A TRUE STORY

Justin always thought that if he "huffs" markers in small doses, just every once in a while, it will cause little or no damage to his brain cells. Maybe, maybe not. We're all different, so you never know when something dangerous will happen to you. Huffing may make you high for a few minutes, but it can damage your brain for a whole lot longer.

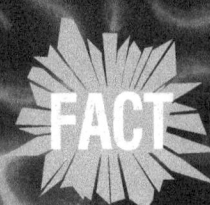

DRUGS MESS WITH YOUR BRAIN'S WIRING AND SIGNALS.

QUIZ

Some drugs affect the brain because their chemical structures are similar to natural brain chemicals called:

A. Neurons
B. Axons
C. Neurotransmitters
D. Dendrites

What is NOT true about "bath salts," often sold in head shops?

A. They can cause intense cravings similar to what methamphetamine users experience.
B. They usually contain some type of stimulant drug along with other unknown ingredients.
C. They are really only dangerous if snorted or injected.
D. They have sent hundreds of people to the emergency room.

Salvia is a herb that can make you:

A. Feel a surge of connectedness to what's around you
B. Experience hallucinations and emotional swings
C. Feel detached and less able to interact with what's going on
D. Both b and c
E. Both a and b

ANSWERS: **C.** Neurotransmitters. **C.** Bath salts, often contain amphetamine-like chemicals including mephedrone, which can put users at risk for an overdose. While snorting or injecting "bath salts" are linked to the most serious health problems including death, taking them orally can also be dangerous. These synthetic stimulants can cause chest pains, increased blood pressure, increased heart rate, agitation, hallucinations, extreme paranoia, and delusions. **D.** Both b and c

TOPIC
Treatment

REHAB?

Does treatment really work? Why do people come and go so much?

It takes time to recover from addiction—not only for the brain to re-adjust, but to make lifestyle changes to avoid drugs. Think how hard it is for people trying to lose weight—they try different diets, exercise for a while, lose a few pounds only to gain them back...until they can make lasting changes to keep the weight off. Same with quitting drugs—it may take several rounds of treatment before it sticks.

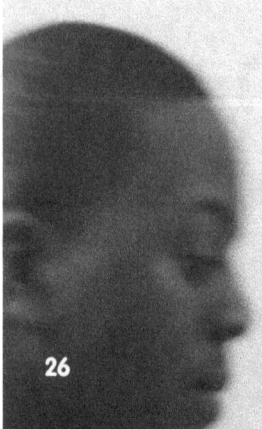

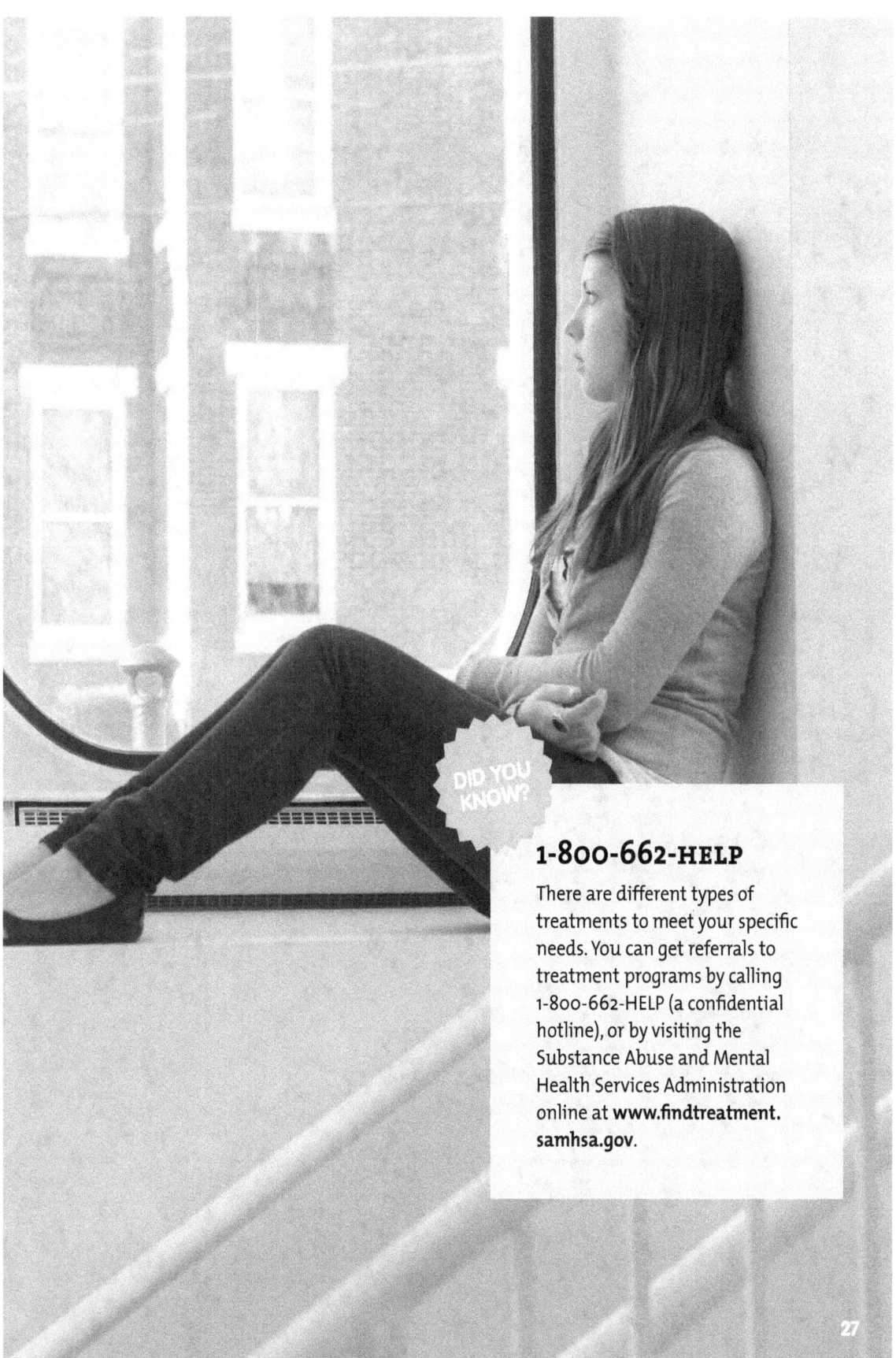

DID YOU KNOW?

1-800-662-HELP

There are different types of treatments to meet your specific needs. You can get referrals to treatment programs by calling 1-800-662-HELP (a confidential hotline), or by visiting the Substance Abuse and Mental Health Services Administration online at **www.findtreatment.samhsa.gov**.

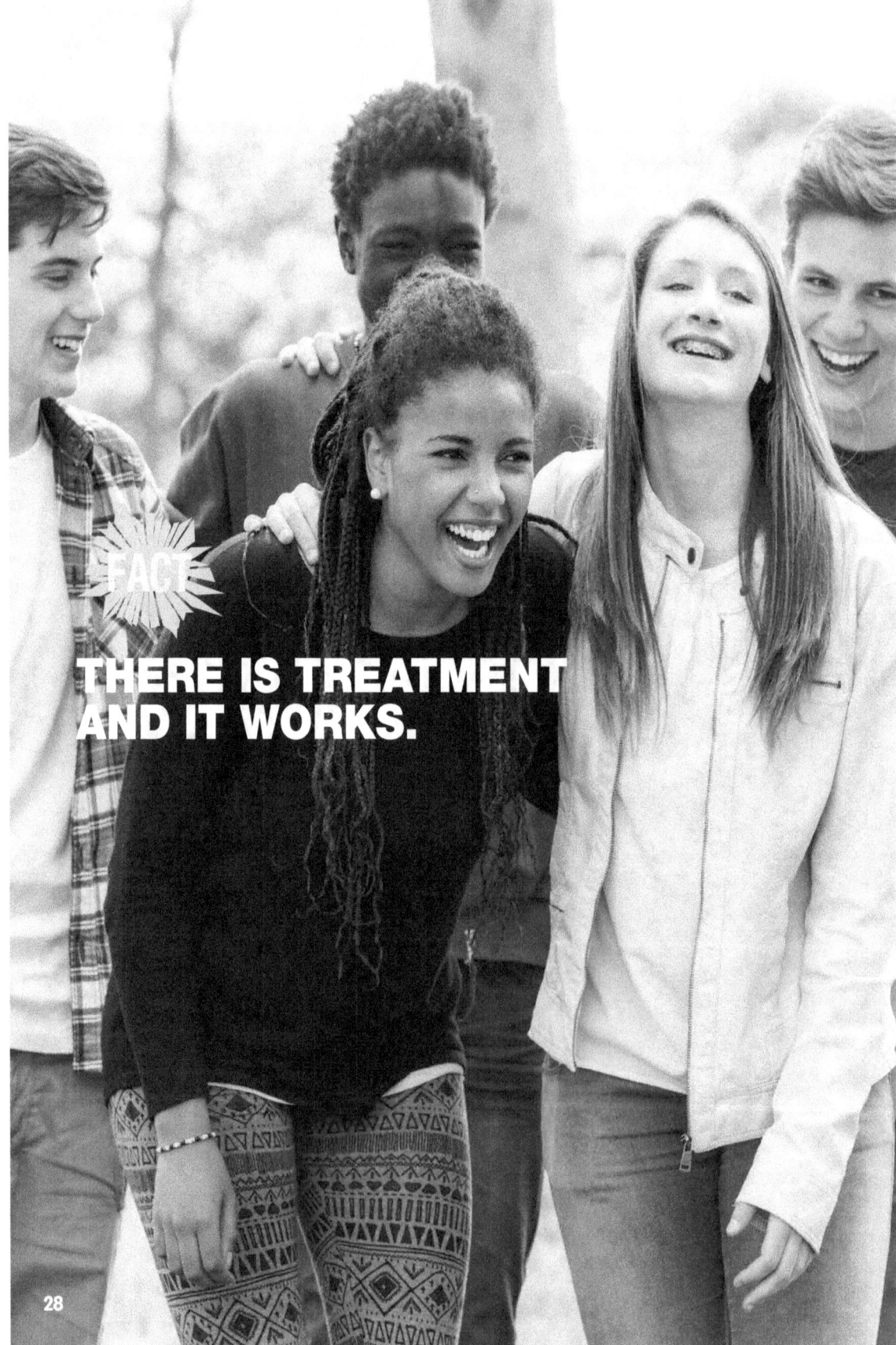

QUIZ

A person who is addicted to drugs...

A. Is beyond reach
B. Can be helped with treatment
C. Needs a brain transplant
D. Can easily quit if they want to

ANSWERS: B. Can be helped with treatment

What do YOU think?

We know you have a lot of questions about drugs. We do too, and we'd love to hear from you! So go to our blog at **http://teens.drugabuse.gov/blog** and let us know what you think—and thanks for sharing!

We also have National Drug Facts Week[SM] (NDFW) each year that helps teens *shatter the myths* about drugs and drug abuse. NDFW includes local school and community events and Drug Facts Chat Day, a live, online chat held between high school students and NIDA scientists. Go to **http://www.teens.drugabuse.gov/national-drug-facts-week** to learn about events in your area. If you have a question about drugs that you haven't seen answered anywhere else, you might be able to find it in the Drug Facts Chat Day transcript (you can find the link on the NDFW website above).

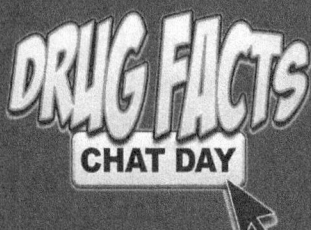

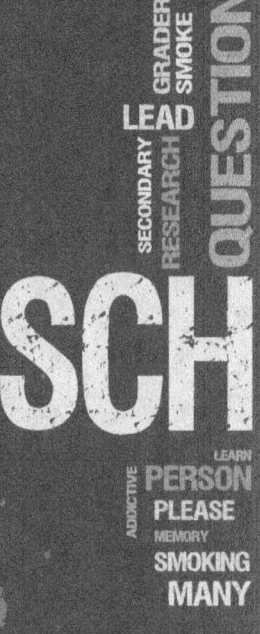

Here are some popular questions we've answered:

- How many young people are addicted to drugs?
- What's the most commonly abused drug by teens?
- Can drugs make you mentally ill?
- What drug is the most addictive?
- Is smoking marijuana more harmful than smoking cigarettes?

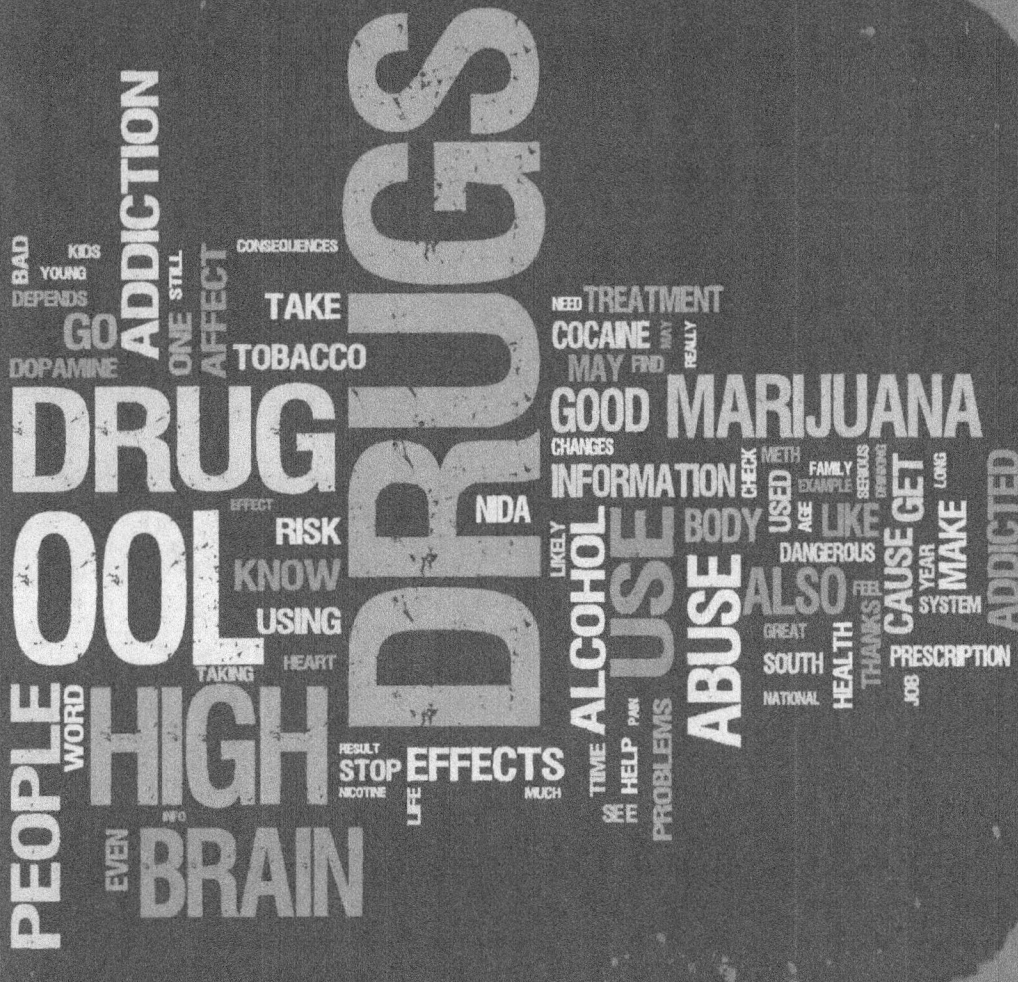

www.ingramcontent.com/pod-product-compliance
Lightning Source LLC
Chambersburg PA
CBHW082124220526
45472CB00009B/2295